PREGNANCY
for First Time
MOMS
What They Don't Tell You

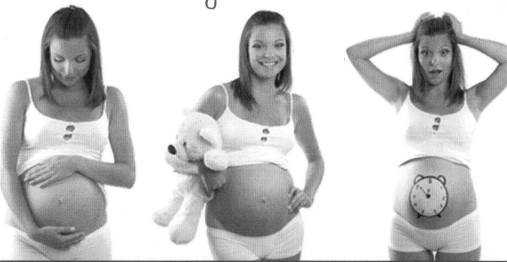

DARELL SPICE

Pregnancy for First-Time Moms

What They Don't Tell You

By Darell Spice

Letter from the Author: I would like to take this opportunity to thank you for purchasing my book, "Pregnancy for First-Time Moms: What They Don't Tell You". My goal in writing this book is to inform and educate others about pregnancy. There are so many women, going through pregnancy for the first time, that have many unanswered questions about their different experiences. This book gives some insight for different situations that may arise. The goal is to ease those concerns so the pregnancy is a more enjoyable experience. I hope this book is a help and thank you again. I have added two BONUS Books at the end of the Book. *"The 10 foods to Avoid during Pregnancy,"* and *"Understanding Postnatal Depression."* I look to always improve my books for my readers. Thank you all for your feedback you have provided me! Please enjoy this book. I hope it may add value to pregnancy and life!

PREGNANCY
for First Time
MOMS

What They Don't Tell You

DARELL SPICE

Table of Contents

BONUS Book: Ten Foods to Avoid during Pregnancy

BONUS Book: Understanding Postnatal Depression

Introduction

I want to thank you and congratulate you for downloading the book, **"Pregnancy for First-Time Moms; What They Don't Tell You".**

This book contains proven steps and strategies on how to make it those wonderful nine months of pregnancy knowing everything that you can expect, even the things that the doctor, family, and friends don't warn you about.

Thanks again for downloading this book, I hope you enjoy it!

Chapter 1

Motherhood Nine Months Ahead

Becoming a mother for the first time is one of the most incredible feelings in the world. But before you get to that point you must carry baby for nine months. Those nine months are filled with a variety of memorable events, along with some that you would probably rather forget. Nonetheless, they are all worth it the first moment that you meet that precious soul that you carried inside of you for so long. Pregnancy is a fun and amazing journey.

As a woman with child, you can expect to go to the doctor often to make sure that baby is growing as it should and to ensure that there are no problems that need doctor intervention. These regular doctor visits help ensure that you and your baby are getting the best care needed during this time. During the first trimester you make visits to the doctor once every month in most cases. Sometimes the doctor will want you to come in more often if you are expecting multiples or have other problems with your pregnancy. The second trimester stays pretty much the same concerning your visits, except these three months are filled with a lot of testing. In the third trimester things change and you are preparing to deliver your new precious bundle of joy. Your doctor will monitor you and Baby closely during these last months of pregnancy.

As you go along in your pregnancy there will be a lot of people who have such great things to tell you to expect. There is nothing like the pregnancy glow that comes. You certainly are going to enjoy every single flutter of your baby inside of you. The first time that the heartbeat is heard it is a tender moment, and the ultrasound is the first picture of your new child. These experiences make your pregnancy very real and special. These moments are just some of the things that onlookers are so eager to tell you.

 But are the nine months of pregnancy all glorious and wonderful? Most people would have you think this way, but the truth of the matter is they are not. You are going to experience tons of weird and strange things while you are pregnant, and most of the time no one tells you about these things. When you are pregnant for the first time many things happen that unless you know what to expect, you may think that something is wrong. This isn't to say that pregnancy is horrible, because it is not. Being pregnant is a part of life. It is a special time, an amazing feeling to know that you have created life and are now nourishing it into this world.

This is the purpose of this guide: to provide soon-to-be mothers with the information that you need and should know while you are pregnant. You can learn the good, the bad   and   the   ugly.

There are so many small, silly things that come along with pregnancy, and sometimes even rather gross things. It is those things that people seem to forget to tell you.

Without further ado, continue reading to learn those secrets about pregnancy that you really want to know. Learn the secrets of all of the trimesters of pregnancy, as well as a few things that you should know about delivering your baby and what to expect after the fact.

Pregnancy is one of the most thrilling times of your life. It is also a time in your life when there is going to be so many amazing changes that you will experience. Now it is time to learn them all and prepare for this nine-month ride.

Chapter 2

First Trimester: What They Don't Tell You

The first trimester of pregnancy is really an introduction period for your body and the new baby. Much is going on inside you and changes are happening to make room for the baby to grow. And get all of the nutrients it needs to mature into a full term fetus. The first trimester is the moment of conception up to the 12th week, or the 3rd month. For many women this is the most difficult trimester of them all. Your body is making a lot of adjustments.

The experience during first trimester varies for all women. You may not feel pregnant or then again you may feel very pregnant. Some women say that they have a full feeling inside of their stomachs from the very moment they conceive. Others even swear they know the exact moment that the baby was conceived. While there are no medical tests that can confirm a pregnancy this early, it is very much possible for a woman to have this type of experience.

 It is hard to know for sure what you will experience or how intense your experience will be. Heartburn, morning sickness, being uncomfortable and nauseated -- these are all things that are commonly experienced by pregnant women during the first trimester.

What is the truth of the matter? Sometimes these experiences can be very difficult, and even if you have experienced them before pregnancy, these experiences are more intense during pregnancy. Heartburn is maximized 10 times over; your body is hot and you feel bloated. Even the smell of water makes you want to run to the bathroom to vomit. Morning sickness, even when you do not actually vomit, can cause pure misery. And, has anyone warned you about dry heaves? These are a few of the common experiences that occur during your first trimester.

Morning Sickness & More

Morning sickness should really have a new name because it is very misleading. It is sickness all right, but it does not discriminate and it causes trouble in more than just the morning. For some pregnant women morning sickness can be absolutely horrible, disrupting life in every single way. These women cannot stay out of the bathroom, and sometimes it is not that they are throwing up, but that they feel as if they want to 24 hours a day. It is not a pretty picture that we are painting here, and that is because there is nothing pretty about morning sickness. It can occur morning, noon and night, and sometimes it occurs during all three and never goes away. A package of saltines on hand to bite on when morning sickness strikes is the new-mom secret. A Sprite or ginger ale can also do the trick to ease your sickness. Do not think that you will only have mild nausea in the morning and it will all go away. This is one of the marks of pregnancy and most women will have it. And, chances are that it is going to be pretty severe for the first trimester. If you do not experience morning sickness, or if it is something that you experience only in mild form, then you are very lucky.

If you normally do not go to the bathroom very often, then get ready for that to change after pregnancy. The bathroom is your best friend during your pregnancy.

Going there will be something that you have to do often! As soon as you wash your hands and get comfortable on the couch, you will have to go again. There's a lot of pressure with a baby sitting on your bladder, even if it does only weigh a half an ounce. The problem with frequent urination is that it doesn't go away until the pregnancy is over. In fact, the bigger baby gets, the worse the problem gets, too.

Heartburn, Acne & More

Heartburn is also something that you probably will experience during the first trimester. It is one of the most common side effects during pregnancy. Women who are pregnant with multiples report that the heartburn is even worse. However, most women with child will experience heartburn, and it really burns. It is a good idea to go ahead and get a bottle of Tums and expect to chew them like candy. You can drink water to help ease heartburn as well.

Even if you have been lucky enough to have never had a pimple before in your life, the hormonal changes with pregnancy may very well bring on an outbreak. For many women in their first trimester acne is a big concern. Many pregnant women fear using the products sold over the counter to get rid acne, scared that it will harm the baby. However, there are numerous home remedies for acne available that are perfectly safe for both mom and baby, while also being effective at eliminating acne breakouts. Some women experience no breakouts, some a few pimples and zits, and other women have full blown breakouts, and again, this is not something that anyone can determine ahead of time. If it does affect you, the key is to be prepared and ready to treat. If you do want to help keep your skin looking its very best, make sure that you wash the face twice per day, using a gentle soap or a mild cleanser. Follow up with a moisturizer to keep the skin soft. You can also talk to your doctor about acne treatments if you do not want to use those that are sold over the counter. Your doctor can give you many other tips and tricks to help combat acne as well.

You are going to be tired. Really tired. No matter how much you sleep it will never seem as if you have had enough. And, when you are awake you are probably not going to be jumping up and down and full of energy. Pregnancy takes a lot out of you. Make plans to settle down just a little bit, compared to your normal activities, that is. While you do not have to sit in the house and do nothing but protect your belly all day, you do need to make a few exceptions, avoid a few things and prepare for those days when staying in bed. You are not going to be getting a lot of sleep in nine months, and you are going to want it. So, go ahead and take advantage of it now, and sleep in when you can and put some of the normal activities to the side. The most important things that you can do right now is take care of your body and the new baby that is growing inside of you, and one of the things that you can do is get the extra sleep that you need.

An Emotional Roller Coaster

Aside from those kinds of changes, expect your emotions to be up and down. Many would suspect you were bipolar if they did not know you were pregnant. The smallest of things can cause an emotional meltdown -- and we do mean a meltdown. Uncontrollable crying isn't uncommon, and expect to be ultra-sensitive. You may cry over every single movie that you see, and something as crazy as getting a hamburger with a pickle on it can send you into frenzy. Your body is going through many changes. It isn't your fault; it is all of those hormones that your body is accumulating.

Mood changes are very common. One minute you are fine and the next you are not. It is just a part of pregnancy. This is first seen in the first trimester, but it is one of those things that continue throughout the entire pregnancy.

Here are a few other very important things that you need to know about pregnancy in the first trimester.

1.   You will also worry about everything. What if you fall while walking down the street? What if something is wrong with the baby? Are you going to be a good mother? Will you produce enough breast milk? What are the best diapers? While seemingly irrational to the non-pregnant brain, prepare to worry about the smallest, sillier of things as if they were a major life decision. Just remember, this too shall pass. It is not uncommon for pregnant women to worry about everything. It is a new experience and there is a lot that is going on inside of your body, after all.

2.   During the first trimester you might also notice veins in your body that you have never noticed before. This is not uncommon and many women experience this. Whether in your arms or legs, veins seem to pop out of nowhere.

3.   Noticing that your legs are a little hairier than they usually are, or that your hair is back the day after you shave? Again this is something that you should plan for and prepare for, because for most pregnant women it happens. Pregnancy is one of the healthiest times in the world, as long as you take care of yourself, and this means that hair (everywhere on the body) is growing rapidly. The hair on top of your head will also have this same effect. If you have thin hair, ordinarily expect to get a totally new mane that you will absolute love.

Your Doctor Visits

There is little change that comes during the first trimester physically, and chances are that most people will not even realize that you are pregnant. Although they say that you cannot feel baby move around until many weeks into the pregnancy, it is very much possible to feel butterflies in the stomach, which is the baby. This is just something that you know when you feel it. It is certainly a feeling like nothing else in this world.

The doctor will see you once a month during the first trimester, and sometime during the 8th week he will listen for a heartbeat. This is an amazing sound to hear. Some doctors will record it for you if you would like, and this is definitely an amazing memory to have to hold. Your doctor will also give you a due date, a date of conception and a ton of information to take home with you and read, including pregnancy magazines.

Most moms would tell you to read these books and learn as much as you can, and you should. But, at the same time, remember that you need to give yourself leeway and rarely does a pregnancy happen just as they predict in those magazines. Every woman will have her own unique experience and this is all a part of the enjoyment of being pregnant. Learn from the books and magazines and do all that you can to abide by the rules and the tips that they offer. But at the same time, do not make the mistake of thinking that everything is going to happen just like it says in those books.

And, another tip, do not throw all of those advertisements away. You are still new to being pregnant, and you are still unaware of just what it means to be a new mom. But, the pregnancy companies out there do and they are ready to help you out. Baby will drink a massive amount of formula, and at a cost of about $30 a can, this can get expensive quickly. Add to that the cost of diapers and you have a very expensive new life forming inside of you. It is all worth it, but you might as well take advantage of all of the help that you can get. Many of those advertisements that you see in magazines are for baby clubs. It is a good idea to go ahead and join them now. You will get plenty of full size products in the mail and lots of extra goodies, too. This can include diaper bags, bottles, wipes, formula, birth announcements, photos and more. You never know what kind of offers that you will find inside, but join all of the clubs that you can!

Chapter 3

The Second Trimester: What They Don't Tell You

By the time the second trimester rolls around (month four) you are getting over the newness of being pregnant. You may be starting to get a little bit of a pooch in the stomach indicating that baby is growing inside. This is certainly exciting. For some people the morning sickness has ceased, but not for everyone. The second trimester lasts from weeks 16 through 24. It is a three-month period when it really starts to 'sink in' that you are with child and soon to become a mommy.

But, from this point forward you can expect the physical changes to take place rapidly. You will go from no-show to big belly in no time flat, once the second trimester rolls around. One of the changes that can be expected during the second trimester is a lack of concentration. You may seem to be unable to focus on much of anything, and sometime you might find yourself saying some pretty off the wall stuff. Don't worry, because almost all pregnant women do it.

As mentioned above, your body starts to change physically a great deal during the second trimester of pregnancy. You will probably want to get some maternity clothes very soon. While you may not need them exactly at the start of the second trimester, the clothes will be needed before very many weeks pass. Buying maternity clothes is a lot of fun and there are tons of great maternity stores where you can shop to get all of you great items.

Sex & Your Pregnancy

Now, are you ready for this? If you want, go get your husband and let him read this one to you. The smile on his face is going to tell you what he has read. While you are in the second trimester, expect your sex drive to be in overdrive. You won't be able to get enough, and it is certainly true that pregnancy sex is very intense with even more exciting orgasms. If the doctor is the one that told you this, you might be a little embarrassed, but not knowing that it is coming can also throw you for a loop.

With the increased desire in sex, it also must be said that when you are pregnant you will worry about sex and whether or not it will hurt the baby. Is your husband well endowed and you're afraid it is going to hit baby in the head? Will the force of sex cause you to miscarry or to go into labor early? While all of these things are certainly there for you to worry about, it is all without reason. Sex does not hurt the baby. It is all in your head. It is not possible for his organ to reach the baby, and for most couples sex is completely safe and encouraged.

Some women want to have a lot of sex during the second trimester, but some women could care less if they ever have it. This is not something that anyone will know before it happens, but know that it could go either way. If you are one of the women who do not want to have sex during this period of time, it is okay. Do not panic. Your drive for sex will come back before you know it and things will be back to normal in no time at all. And, when it does come back, expect that sex drive to be in full swing.

More 2nd Trimester Pregnancy Information

Expect to really pack on the weight during the second trimester. In fact, you might notice that you have gained a pound or two every time that you stand on the scale. And this is okay. This is an important time for baby, and he or she is growing rapidly. That weight is all a part of a normal pregnancy and should be welcomed. As long as you are eating right, there is nothing to worry about! People will start touching your belly a lot during this time, and you will probably be in the mirror a lot admiring the changes that your body is going through. Your breasts may start to feel more round and firm during this time and they may also start slightly growing in size. Most women are very happy about this pregnancy change.

By the second trimester you will regain some of your energy, but do be prepared for some pretty massive cravings. There is absolutely nothing in this world like the cravings that a pregnant woman has. No matter how unusual or odd they may seem to the pregnant individual, the pregnant women must have them or else. Expect to crave something, unless you have an all-around top-notch diet going on already.

Pregnant women also commonly experience uncontrollable sweating, especially during the second trimester. This is something that many pregnant women complain about, especially at night when they are sleeping. If you are bothered by this problem you may be dehydrated. Again you need to eat and drink for two, so your body needs extra vitamins and nutrients to make it. Make sure that you are drinking plenty of water while you are pregnant and staying hydrated.

Many pregnancy women also experience bleeding gums. This is something that can actually start before the second trimester, but for most it is within these months that it occurs. For most women the problem ceases after pregnancy, but if you already have gum problems or diseases or other oral health concerns you may want to speak with your dentist about the problem. It is usually not a big concern.

Back Pain during Pregnancy

Back pain is one of those things that almost all women experience. It is usually in the lower back that most of the pain is experienced, but sometimes it can extend beyond the lower back. It can be very severe for many, and sometimes it puts them in bed because it is so bad. There is so much added pressure on the body that you can only imagine the pain in the back. There are a few things that you can do to ease or minimize the back pain, but do expect it to come. If you are one of the lucky ones that do not have back pain with pregnancy, this is something else that you should be thankful for because it is very common.

First of all, practice good posture. This will help you now and as your pregnancy continues. When you are sitting straight in a chair, it will support your back and this can minimize the pain. Go ahead and invest in one of those pregnancy pillows. They are relatively affordable and you will get tons of use out of it since you can use it even after baby is born. You can use the pillow to place between your legs to help ease the pain you feel in your back, and the pillow is also great to lay your head on for elevation and support, too.

It is also a really good time to go ahead and invest in three to four good pairs of shoes and put those that you normally wear in the back of the closet. One of the biggest causes of back pain during pregnancy is wearing shoes that are not supportive. Make sure that you aren't wearing while you are pregnant as this increases the pain that you will feel and can cause harm to the baby if you were to fall. Your shoes should be flat and supportive. There are some brands of shoes made specifically for pregnancy, and you may find those shoes to be your best bet.

This is also the perfect time to ask your significant other for a nice back rub or a foot rub. While a massage is amazing any time, when your body is aching during pregnancy it is even more flattering, and you will enjoy every second of it.

Chapter 4

Changes with the Breasts

Expect your boobs to start changing really quickly after learning of your pregnancy, and those changes are going to occur the entire nine months that you are with child. In fact, tender, sore breasts may be one of the signs that alert you to the pregnancy in the first place. The changes with the breast do not stop after this initial period, and there are a variety of things that you can expect to happen during those nine months.

First of all, understand that your breasts are going to feel...strange. They may feel soft and perky one day and the next not quite so welcoming to oncoming traffic. You will know that your breasts are there, even if you've never really given them much thought before. As you go along in your pregnancy, the breasts can become quite large and heavy. The further that you get in the pregnancy the more changes that will occur and the changes will be far more noticeable as well. Many women feel that their breasts are heavier than usual when they are pregnant and this is especially true during the latter months.

Your breasts are going to get bigger, so go ahead and plan to buy new bras. The increase in bust size that will be experienced varies from new mommy to new mommy, but some women increase three to four cup sizes or more. You want to take the time to choose good supporting bras during this time. There are many bras made specifically to handle those bigger than average breasts.

Those changes will also affect your nipples; so if you look down and they are bigger, darker, fuller or otherwise more noticeable, do not be alarmed. Another possible thing that you will experience while pregnant, but not to be worried about, is small, pin-sized bumps forming around the nipples. This is something that many women experience and it is all a part of the hormones that are causing it.

During the last few trimesters of pregnancy as your body prepares to welcome your new bundle of joy, expect colostrum to leak from the breasts. For women who are not aware that this will happen, it can be pretty scary, but it is nothing serious and pretty normal actually. Colostrum leakage is actually a good sign that indicates that your body is in check with baby and preparing for the delivery, as it should be during this time.

The amount of leakage that you will experience will vary, however, so do not be alarmed if you find yourself leaking larger quantities than expected. Some women report small leakage now and again while other women report flooding bras. There are breast pads available that help catch the leakage. Go ahead and buy them now, Mommy, because the leaking of milk once baby arrives is also going to send you running to the maternity store to pick them up.

Colostrum is the breast milk that baby will feed upon during the first day or two of life. It isn't actually milk, but rather a special protein-filled liquid that Baby needs when he is born. Your body begins producing the colostrum several months before Baby is due.

When baby does arrive, as we just mentioned you could expect milk to leak out of the breasts. Again, there is no way to determine how much you will leak, but do prepare for a worst case scenario because many women report major leaking a few days after baby is born. Your breasts will be larger, and probably firmer. They are also going to shrink eventually, so do prepare for this.

Chapter 5

Carpal Tunnel Syndrome

Carpal tunnel syndrome is a condition that can be experienced even if you are not pregnant. However, it seems to be that those nine months can cause an onset of the condition quicker than anything. It is during the 2nd and 3rd trimesters that carpal tunnel syndrome can really affect the woman. For most it is something that goes away after the baby is born. Carpal tunnel syndrome causes numbness, tingling and pain in the hands and the arms.

There are different severities of carpal tunnel syndrome, and for those women who are affected it will do so in a different way. For some women it is so severe that they drop things.

Carpal tunnel syndrome occurs when pressure is placed on the median nerve. This nerve is found in the wrist, and is formed by the bones in the wrist, or the carpals, as well as ligament. The nerve controls movement of the thumb as well as all of the feeling that goes to it. When this added pressure is placed on the thumb it causes the problems due to the increased sensitivity.

If problems with the condition become severe, it is a good idea to talk to your doctor. He may want to intervene with some sort of treatment. If you do not want any type of doctor intervention and feel that the problem is not that serious, there are several things that you can do to remedy the problem on your own.

First and foremost you want to try to learn what it is that you are doing that causes aggravation. Once you learn what this problem is you can stop doing this as much as possible, which will help minimize the experiences that you are feeling. Wearing your arm or hand in a sling at night to maintain a neutral position is also an idea that can help minimize the pain. Some women do this trick during the day as well and, as long as you are able to move about the way you need, there is nothing wrong with that.

When you are at work try to minimize the use of your hands as much as possible, and make adjustments to the height of your chair and desk to accommodate the pain. Sometimes moving your hand in another direction is all that it takes to alleviate the pain. It is also important to remember that you need to take breaks, and perhaps more frequently than you would if you were not pregnant. A final tip is to sleep with your feet higher than your head and spread out wider than usual. Pillows can help do the trick here.

Chapter 6

Pregnancy Tests – There are Many

We are not talking about the pregnancy test that confirmed you were indeed with child. We are talking about the many different tests that will need to be performed during your pregnancy. There are several of them, and each is just as important as the next in ensuring that your baby is healthy. Expect these tests and prepare ahead for them. All new moms must endure them and just remember that they are all for the best of your bundle of joy.

Gynecologist Exam

This is one of the first exams that you will take, and there are several things that take place during the exam. A pap smear is likely to be one of the things that are performed during the exam. This test checks for signs of cervical cancer, something very important to know when you are pregnant. This is just one of many tests that are performed during the exam. The doctor will also check the cervix and measure its size. A feel of the stomach is also something that you can expect. This exam is likely to take place at all visits that you make to the doctor during the course of your pregnancy.

Ultrasounds

When you are pregnant, those ultrasounds are something to which you will look forward. You probably will not require an ultrasound for a few weeks of the pregnancy if you are having a normal pregnancy, but there are many reasons the doctor may order one. If you want to know the sex of the baby, this is something that you can elect to learn at about five months of gestation. The purpose of the ultrasounds is to make sure that the baby is growing, as he or she should be, that his head size is correct, and to check for possible problems.

Blood Tests

Be prepared to be poked with a needle – a lot. There are assortments of blood tests that are needed when you are pregnant, and these tests check for various problems with the baby and the pregnancy. Having these tests can prevent a lot of problems with the pregnancy, so it is important they are done. It is likely that the doctor will perform a stud test on you on the initial visit, and this also includes a test for HIV. Even if you are in a monogamous relationship it is important to know this status to protect the unborn baby.

Blood Glucose Test

For most pregnant women, a blood glucose test isn't a very pleasant experience. This test checks for diabetes in mom and baby. Even women who were not diabetic before pregnancy have an increased risk during those nine months, and it is imperative to identify the problem as soon as possible. Drinking an orange glucose drink very quickly is the first step of this test. The drink isn't the worst tasting thing in the world, but then again it isn't the best, especially when you are pregnant and already have a full stomach. Expect this test to be taken between 24 and 28 weeks of pregnancy. All women must take this test.

These are just some of the many different tests that you will need to take during your pregnancy. If you have a normal pregnancy, there will be far less testing. If not, or there are concerns or it is a multiple birth, expect there to be more tests on a more frequent basis.

Chapter 7

Third Trimester Changes: What to Expect

The 3rd trimester begins at week 28 and lasts until week 40 when you will give birth. The pregnancy is almost over and the time for baby's arrival is quickly nearing. By this time, you're ready to meet your baby, and you are probably becoming tired of pregnancy. Especially during the latter weeks, no one tells you how ready you will be for it to be over. You just want to have the baby, see your feet again and tie your own shoes. How you miss bending over and sleeping normally!The last trimester is enough, and, fortunately, the time is almost ended.

If you're due on March 25th, don't actually expect to have your baby on this date. Do not make birth announcements, t-shirts and all of that with this date on it simply because your ob/gyn tells you that is the due date. Few women actually deliver on this actual due date. Most women deliver before their actual due dates, but some women carry their baby longer. Generally speaking the doctor will not allow a woman to go past her 42nd week, so prepare for a C-section in that case.

At the start of your 3rd trimester your baby has grown quite large. He is comparable to the size of an eggplant, and weighs anywhere from one and a half pounds to about two and a half pounds, with a length of about 12.5 to 14.9 inches long. By the time the 3rd trimester ends your baby will weigh anywhere from 5.5 pounds to 9.5 pounds, and measure between 17 and 23 inches in length.

Just as you have experienced many changes throughout the pregnancy, the third trimester is also filled with a number of exciting changes, as well as those that are not so pleasant. But, you are nearing the end now, and the experience is almost over. It is not over just yet, and there are still many great firsts that you have yet to experience. The final trimester is really intense with feelings, and you can be certain there is going to be a lot going on in your world. It isn't easy to prepare to bring a new life into the world, you know, and the body is working overtime in order to be able to do that.

Shortness of breath is one of those things that will probably affect your in the 3rd trimester of your pregnancy. This is caused by the weight of the baby and the various pregnancy hormones that are stimulating the brain and the lungs. You may feel as if you are short of breath or may even need to take deeper breaths. There is nothing wrong with you, and this is another one of those common pregnancy concerns. If you already have asthma or other breathing problems, let your doctor know. You may also want to go to the doctor if the shortness of breath seems to be getting worse or if you cannot control the breathing patterns after a few minutes.

Dizziness is another complaint that a large number of pregnant women have in common. After an activity, you find yourself dizzy or faint as you sit in your favorite chair at home, looking at the TV. Dizziness is caused when blood pressure changes and by the various pregnancy hormones. Baby is pretty big at this point, and the added pressure that is being placed on the body can also be responsible for the dizzy spells that you are having. There are actually quite a few things that you can do to minimize this concern, including eating healthy, drinking plenty of water and wearing loose clothing. Make sure that you do not skip meals and that you are increasing the portion of food that you are eating. Do not forget that you are eating for two people, so it is okay to eat more. Make sure that you are also snacking between meals, and eating healthy snacks at that

Other ways to prevent dizziness during pregnancy are to stand slowly and do not stand in the same position for long periods of time.

Bladder leakage is very common during the third trimester of pregnancy. Many pregnant women choose to wear a light pad or a panty liner just for this reason alone. Something as simple as laughing or coughing can cause you to leak a small amount of fluid. No, this doesn't mean that you have overactive bladder and you do not need to make an appointment with the doctor to get a medication, unless this is really severe. Again, this is caused by the weight of the baby sitting on your bladder and a concern that almost all pregnant women have.

The third trimester, especially the 8th and 9th month, is usually spent absolutely miserably. Your feet are swollen, your hands are swollen and you just cannot get comfortable, no matter what it is you do. You can't sit or stand or even lie in the bed these days. You are ready to have the baby and may even be willing to try some of those tricks in old wives' tales to pop the bun out of the oven. But do not do this! Your baby is still growing inside of you, and in due time, it is all going to be over and you will miss it.

Braxton Hicks Contractions

For a first-time pregnant woman, all of the various feelings and flutters and changes are certainly very new and exciting, even those that are not quite so pleasant. At the end of the day, these experiences are all a part of the amazing journey to life. The first time that you feel Braxton Hicks contractions is something that you will never forget. Almost 90% of pregnant women will experience these contractions during the final trimester of their pregnancies, and since it is something that you have never experienced before you may think that it is the real thing. But trust that these contractions are nothing compared to the real thing. These contractions are not actual contractions signaling that baby is ready to come; they are practice contractions that your body uses to help it better prepare for the actual delivery of baby. Braxton Hicks contractions usually start around the 28th week of pregnancy. This kind of contraction feels like a sharp stabbing pain in the uterus, with irregular and unpredictable tightening. If it were a real contraction this tightening and pain would become more intense and the water might break. Remember that you may or may not experience the false contractions, so do not be alarmed either way. Your body is simply in practice mode at the moment. There is a really big job ahead in a matter of a few weeks, you know.

Most women, who are pregnant for the first time finds themselves in the labor and delivery ward for Braxton Hicks contractions, so if you make the same mistake, do not feel so bad. You are eager, and this is all so new to you. After all you wouldn't want to sit at home and have the baby while watching your favorite soap operas, so it is better to be safe than to be sorry! Make sure that you do not simply assume that it is time and rush to the hospital. Call your doctor, and do not panic. In most cases they can tell if it is the false labor or the real deal and can give you the guidance and advice needed.

Chapter 8

More Pregnancy Secrets No One Tells You

We hope that you have gained a lot of information that you did not already know about your pregnancy and are now preparing adequately. Pregnancy is an amazing journey, and, when you know everything that is probably going to happen, it can be an even easier journey for you to make. However, we are still not done and there are a lot of other pregnancy secrets that no one ever seems to tell you but you still must know. If you want to know the rest of those secrets, keep reading.

Touchy Feely Kind of World

It is up to you as to how you will react, but go ahead and start planning it now: People are going to touch your belly. Yes, you can expect all of your family and your friends to do it, and that is annoying enough. (If you don't think so now, just wait. You soon will understand.) But what is really, really bone chilling is that it is not just family and friends who will want to touch the baby belly. The ladies in the supermarket will simply need to put their hands on the belly. Every kid that you encounter when you are shopping is going to touch your belly, or at least ask if they can. Heck, even the mailman might see the belly and feel the desire to touch it. People come out of nowhere to touch a pregnant belly and they could care less to whom that belly is attached. It is just something about that pregnancy belly that people find irresistible. You can politely ask people not to do it, but if you are like most moms you will just suck it up and go with it. It's kind of nice to be fussed about after all.

People Love to Talk

These is really no way to know what will come out of the mouths of some people upon learning that you are pregnant, so do not let anything that you hear surprise you. Sometimes, it is information that is very much unwanted, but it is all given to you with the best of intentions, in most cases. Be prepared for people to tell you things that you should be doing differently, giving you stories of how they did things and so much more. It is just a part of being pregnant, and yet another one of those things that everyone goes through while she is with child. Being prepared to hear some pretty off-the-wall statements can make dealing with them easier.

You will also want to prepare to be called "Mom" or "Mommy" by everyone. Kids love to do this, but adults are also in on it, too. This one isn't so bad, but it might come as a shock to hear it from some people, if you are not at least prepared to hear it

It is kind of nice to be called a mom, but the real treat comes when your baby says it the first time!

Stretch Marks

You have probably been waiting to see those two words this whole guide, wondering why you have yet to see any mention. But do not worry. We haven't forgotten them. We still look at them every single day so there is always that constant reminder there, even if we wanted to forget. People will tell you a lot about stretch marks. Every person has a different tale to tell: how to prevent them or how lucky she was not to get them. It is true that not all pregnant women get stretch marks, but for most women it is impossible to prevent them. If you are one of the lucky people for whom this is not an issue, you can thank your lucky stars for that. Stretch marks occur on the stomach, the arms and the legs, and oftentimes on the beasts, too. They occur due to the increase in the size, which stretches the skin, in such a short period of time. Stretch marks are often nice to see and they have a blue, red or purplish color. African American and Hispanic woman, as well as those of other dark skinned tones, are more likely to develop stretch marks and they are usually darker and deeper on these skin tones. There is not a lot that you can do about stretch marks. Watching what you eat so you do not gain a ton of extra weight is one step. Investing in a good cocoa butter lotion and using it on a regular basis can also help.

What's That Smell?

Have you ever wondered what it is like to be a drug-sniffing dog that has such a heightened sense of smell it can detect the faintest whiff of something? Well, we haven't either, but that is pretty much what it is like to be pregnant. You can smell everything and it is really intense. Many times you will find yourself asking, "What's that smell?" only to have other people tell you that they smell nothing. That is impossible, you think, because you can smell it so well. Your dog-like sense of smell is likely to develop at the very beginning of your pregnancy and continue until you have the baby. Sometimes it is a good thing and sometimes it is not, because you smell it all -- good and bad! Be prepared to have a Wonder Woman sense of smell.

The Movements Are Incredible

The first time that you feel your baby kick is an incredible feeling. It is incredible to feel all of his tiny little flutters and movements. Some people feel them earlier than others, but if you are paying close attention, you will be able to feel them quickly. Be sure that you have your journal ready to write all of these special feelings down.

Document Everything

This is probably not something that you will have any trouble doing. Most pregnant women love to take photos of their baby belly and their pregnancy, but many fail to keep a journal to document those special occasions. Do not assume that you are going to remember everything because you are not. Believe us, Mommy, you have yet to learn. There are tons of themed pregnancy journals and keepsake baby books that let you jot down those special memories and you very well should take advantage and use them. Remembering how you felt that first time you heard the sounds of that tiny heartbeat, how in love you were the moment that you found out, the first ultrasound and glimpse of your baby. These are all things that you want to document, but don't forget those other little and unexpected things. They are just as memorable and certainly a blast to look back upon later in life. Snap pictures until your snapping finger hurts, and keep everything special that happens to you documented in that special journal. You will be glad that you did this later in life.

"I Want It and I Want It NOW"

Ordinarily in life, we see something that we want and we get it when we can. Yes, some things we want more than we want other things, but nonetheless we understand and do what we can to work on getting those items. But when you are pregnant, you will have cravings that are so intense that not getting what you want at that very moment is enough to send you into a tear-filled frenzy for hours on end. The cravings of pregnant women are immense, and sometimes they are also very odd. The body craves what it is lacking in most cases, so if you are eating healthy you are less likely to have those cravings. For most women, though, there will be something that you simply cannot live without and would drive 500 miles to get it. Expect this.

Hemorrhoids

Yep, the real pain in the butt. Hemorrhoids are for old people who aren't eating their Raisin Bran. That notion is incorrect. Anyone can get a hemorrhoid at any age, and when you are pregnant the odds of its happening are even greater. It doesn't matter if you're 20 or 40; pregnancy doubles the risk of hemorrhoids. Again, it is all about the added pressure on the body, the rectal area and the weight of the uterus. Hemorrhoids really hurt, and that pain intensifies while you are pregnant. You may or may not get a hemorrhoid, but it is important to know it is possible. If you have a hemorrhoid, it is difficult to go to the bathroom and it also makes it difficult to sit, lie down or do much of anything else. There are many over-the-counter treatments for hemorrhoids, should you be one of the unlucky ones who develop them. You can also talk to your doctor about treatment options, if you are getting them on a frequent basis, if the over-the-counter products are not working or if you are simply concerned with baby's health and want the expert advice first. You can also help lower the odds of getting a hemorrhoid by eating a well-balanced diet. It isn't just the Raisin Bran that can help with a hemorrhoid; many fruits and vegetables are high in fiber content.

Four Weeks & a Wake-Up

The last month of pregnancy is definitely the hardest. While the last trimester itself is uneasy, it is those last four weeks that seem to make even the calmest, gentlest of people feel as if are going to lose their minds. Prepare to be uneasy all of the time and probably really grumpy and biting the heads off of everyone who so much as speaks to you. Emotions and mood swings are also going to be really high. Remember, all of those hormones are going crazy inside of your body! Everything is going to make you cry, and there may be people who are looking at you with a lot of wonder in their eyes. Ignore them. If they are mothers, they will understand. The last four weeks also seem like an eternity, so expect that to be something that you experience as well. Soon you will be free, but in the meantime prepare yourself and everyone around you for this last month. Once they have been warned, all is fair in pregnancy.

Chapter 9

After Baby: Secrets They Don't Tell You

There is so much that no one tells you about being pregnant, and we hope that all of the chapters inside of this book have helped you learn many of the things of which you otherwise would have been unaware. But, there is still more. There are a ton of things that you should know when you have the baby, too. Your body is not back to normal the minute that you have a baby. This is a major job, as you might expect. Your body has to have the time it needs to recover, which is generally a period of about six weeks. In some cases, the doctor will recommend that you remain on a low activity plan for a period of eight weeks. This all depends upon your exact situation. You will have a postpartum visit before the six-week period and again at the six-week mark. The doctor will give you the green light to go if all is normal. This means that you can go back to work and resume all of your normal activities, including sex. Yes, the husband will be happy about this, if he isn't too tired to do the do now that baby is keeping him up all hours of the day and night.

But there are also a lot of other secrets that you need to know, too. Just as you do not want to be surprised and unprepared while you are carrying baby, you do not want that to happen after the baby makes debut in this world. Take a look at some of the things no one tells you in time.

No Sex & Heavy Bleeding

So many people say that you will bleed after you have a baby, but they fail to tell you that this is not the same kind of blood you experience during a period or under normal circumstances. Some women say they bleed so much they often think they are going to shed all of the blood out of their body. Bleeding very heavily the first few weeks after pregnancy is to be expected, and this is true whether you deliver vaginally or via a C-section. You will probably not be able to use the normal pads that are made for menstrual cycles, so do not try it. The hospital will likely give you a few extra large pads to take home with you and you will also need to buy some of these, too.. You will need plenty of them. And, in case you did not already figure it out, you cannot have sex right after you have the baby, usually for about six weeks. You will be bleeding pretty heavily during this time anyway and trying to adjust to this probably won't bother either of you anyway. When the postpartum visit takes place, the doctor can give you the green light to have sex once again, so do not do it until then. You can potentially damage your organs if you are having sex too early. Again, having a baby causes a lot of stress to the body and it needs time to recover from it all.

Speaking of heavy bleeding, did we also mention that the blood might be a little chunky too? Yes, kind of a nasty thought, but, again, it is one of those things that you will be glad to know ahead of time. It can be pretty freaky to go to the bathroom to see bright red chunks of blood coming out of your vagina, but it is normal and most women will do this.

A Little Sore & Swollen

Again, a statement true whether you have baby naturally or via a C-section: Be prepared for your private parts to be sore and swollen. Look at the things that they have been put through and you can understand why they may be sore and swollen. They are probably going to be pretty ugly, too, so expect these things and it will not be such an overwhelming shock to you to experience.

Normal Is out of the Question

Do not expect to return to normal after having a baby. The real question is "what is normal?" Whatever normal was to you before baby, you no longer know it.. Having a baby changes everything, and you have probably heard this a million times. You will love the new experience that you have but will miss the sleep. You will rush to the crib every time that you can, to simply make sure that your baby is breathing. You will want everything to be perfect, and will probably not even want people to look at the baby, much less touch her.

Postpartum Depression

Postpartum depression is a very serious concern that affects a large number of women after they give birth. Oftentimes referred to as the baby blues, postpartum depression can make that joyous occasion far less exciting. If you are feeling down and out, sad, crying more than usual or not wanting to care for your baby, these are all signs of postpartum depression and getting help from your doctor immediately is something that you should do. Many women feel bad that they are feeling less than adequate as a new mother, but you should not. There is a medical reason for the way that you feel and there is help available. The worst thing that you can do is fail to seek help. This is not a condition that will improve on its own and it will only get worse with time. If you have such feelings, contact your doctor immediately and do not wait for the visit to occur at the six-week period. When you are not in the best of health you cannot take the best care of your baby. It is just as important that you are taking care of yourself.

Your Size Will Stay the Same

Do not expect to shrink back down to your pre-pregnancy size after you pop the baby out. For most women this just does not happen, especially immediately after giving birth. Make sure that you have plenty of larger clothes available for after delivery. And most importantly, make sure that they are comfortable. After giving birth, you are going to be very sore and the last thing that you want is uncomfortable clothes adding to that. Many women still wear their maternity clothes after they have baby because they still fit and this might also be something that you wish to do as well.

Your Breasts Will Shrink & More

You have probably come to love your nice, full breasts that you developed during pregnancy, but like all good things this will come to an end. Women who are breastfeeding will find their breasts to stay large after they have the babies, but if you do not, they will probably resume normal size. Some women do report they are a cup larger or even a cup smaller after birth, so do prepare for your old bras not to fit you anymore.

Your breasts will remain heavy after you give birth and leaking milk from your breasts is something that you can expect to happen. It is a good idea to invest in a good breast pump whether you plan to breastfeed or not. If you are not planning to breastfeed, the milk needs to be pumped and removed from the breasts. Expect breasts to be very sore and also very sensitive during this time.

Poo Poo Platter

Yes, we have to talk about the nasties right now, and you will thank us later for letting you in on this secret, even if it does turn your stomach right now. When you are in labor, expect to let out a little poo. Yes, we are talking about number 2. Your doctor is ready for it, so you should be, too. About 90% of all women will do it during labor. Don't worry about the embarrassment. You won't be concerned during that time and after the miracle of birth you are likely to forget all about it. Of course, if you do want to bring it up and offer the doctor a "Hey, I am sorry for pooing on you," by all means feel free to do that.

Breastfeeding 101: The Doctor Won't Tell You This

You have decided to breastfeed your baby to ensure that he is the healthiest he can be. Give yourself a pat on the back because there is no way to deny that breast is best for baby. Expect that to come with a bit of troubles. It is unusual for mom and a baby to get it down pat the very first time. Latching on is often something that babies have trouble doing, and sometimes it hurts when baby sucks, until you get it right. You are not the only new mom who is struggling to breastfeed, but it will get much easier with time. Once you have gotten the hang of things, you will find that breastfeeding is very relaxing, very enjoyable. It may even send pleasure to the brain and be something that you like. Many women even report that breastfeeding will put them to sleep, but they are also often embarrassed that they find breastfeeding to be such a pleasurable, relaxing experience. But do not be, this is also normal and something that many women experience. As with many of the changes that pregnancy brings, this all has to do with the hormones.

While rare, there have been reports of women who actually have orgasms when they are breastfeeding. If you are one of the women who find this to be enjoyable, do not feel as if there is something wrong with you. There are so many other awesome new moms who are also experiencing the same enjoyment from it as you, and it is a completely natural feeling to have. Do not feel ashamed and certainly do not give up breastfeeding because you think this is weird.

An Overwhelming Need to Protect Your Baby

One look in your baby's eyes will melt your heart and it is at that moment that you have experienced love and now understand its true meaning. You will also have an overwhelming desire to protect your baby in every single way possible. You will hate hearing those tiny little cries, especially when you do not know what to do for your baby. You will want to stop baby from crying as quickly as you possibly can, but not because the noise bothers you, but because it is a signal that something is wrong and this is the last thing that you want for your new baby.

You Will Learn the Cries

What do those cries mean, speaking of a crying baby? Since a baby cannot talk, crying is the one and only way that it has to communicate with you. While the cries might all sound the same at first, it will very quickly turn around and you will be able to identify your baby's cries and just what they mean. No, this is not some sort of magic trick; it is simply a mom trick. Usually those high-pitched cries are those signaling that something is wrong. Always remember that addressing your baby and his cries as quickly as you possible can help to build trust with your child. Feel confident that you will soon learn all of his cries and what they mean. Also, remember that sometimes baby will cry just to be crying. Maybe he is bored; maybe he just doesn't feel good on a particular day. Sometimes all that you can do is be there, hold your baby and do all that you can to comfort her until she is feeling better.

The Love of Becoming a Mother: Cherish Every Moment

Becoming a mother is a feeling, which no words can describe. It is an immense love, an unconditional love, and a special bond that no one can understand except for another mother. The pregnancy is a time that is also very special as you grow the new life inside of you. All of the moments of your pregnancy are not going to be the best, but they are all very much exciting and things that you will never again forget in your life. It is an incredible feeling to carry another life inside of you.

While there are many surprises that will come your way during pregnancy, they are all very much worth the amazing person that you have created. The love between a mother and a child is undeniable and you will begin growing and bonding with your child every single day from this point forward.

The most important thing that no one tells you is to cherish every single day of your pregnancy. It isn't all pleasant and it isn't all enjoyable. But it is a once-in-a-lifetime experience, a miracle in the works. It is pretty amazing to carry another person inside of body and to have the ability to create new life. You will love being a mother, and until you hold your baby in your arms for the first time, it is not a feeling that can be explained. There is nothing like it. The special time that you carry your bundle of joy should be cherished and appreciated because it is all a part of bringing that beautiful baby to life. There isn't anything in this world that could be better than that. Use all of this information to the best of your ability, but, at the end of the day, remember that you are experiencing the miracle of life, and it is something that you should appreciate.

Conclusion

Thank you again for downloading this book!

My goal in creating this book is to give helpful and useful information to help you through your pregnancy. Becoming a mother is one of the most rewarding feelings in the world. And knowing what to expect, helps you to be able to focus on your baby and enjoy your pregnancy. It is my sincerest goal to assist in this process.

So, I would love to know your thoughts on the material and get some feedback. You can do this by taking a few moments and giving my book a review. This information is very helpful for me, in my effort to help others. Whether you thought the book was great or if there was other subject matter that you wish had been included. I look over all my reviews and make changes based on your thoughts and opinions. So please tell me what you think. I would love to know your thoughts, and thanks again!

Bonus Book:

Ten Foods to Avoid During Pregnancy

10 Foods to Avoid During Pregnancy

Pregnancy is an amazing gift a woman can ever have! Being able to conceive a life within is a wonderful experience that can't be explained by words! When pregnant, a woman has to take care of herself intensely for the safety of her growing baby. Food eaten during pregnancy plays an important role in the development of the baby. There are a lot of healthy food options, but there are a few foods that should not be consumed during pregnancy. Read on to find out about the top 10 food items that need to be avoided while being pregnant.

1. Unpasteurized Dairy Products

Dairy products, such as milk and cheese, contain bacteria that cause food-borne illness. So, never consume them if they are not pasteurized. Always read the label to confirm before purchasing. Besides, soft, mold-ripened, blue-veined cheeses, such as brie and camembert, are potential dairy products where bacteria such as listeria grow. Listeria affects the growing fetus and causes developmental problems, so avoid eating soft cheese during pregnancy.

2. Raw Sea Food

Raw seafood, especially shellfish such as oysters, is better avoided as it contains harmful parasites that affect the growing fetus. Also, avoid sushi that has raw fish as one of the ingredients. Though smoked fish should not be eaten, it is still okay to consume them when thoroughly cooked.

3. Fish High in Mercury

Fish is a high source of protein and omega – 3 fatty acids essential during pregnancy. However, certain fish have a high level of mercury that is harmful for the growing fetus. Mercury affects the developing nervous system. So, eliminate big fish like swordfish, shark and marlin totally from your diet. Tuna is good to eat when cooked properly, however, limit the intake.

4. Undercooked Poultry, Meat & Eggs

Pregnant women are more prone to food poisoning and bacterial infections. Undercooked or raw poultry, meat or eggs contain harmful bacteria that cause a mild fever for weeks affecting the growth of the baby. So never, consume these food products unless they are cooked properly and served hot.

5. **Unwashed Vegetables & Fruits**

Make sure you wash fruits and vegetables thoroughly before consuming as they might contain bacteria. Also, avoid eating raw sprouts, as it is difficult to wash away disease-causing bacteria from them. However, cooked sprouts are safe.

6. **Over Consumption of Vitamin A**

Limit the consumption of food containing Vitamin A as it causes birth defects. Vitamin A that is naturally present in fruits and vegetables is good during pregnancy. But avoid liver, as it contains maximum amount of Vitamin A, which is not good. Moreover, a supplement will not be necessary as an average woman gets vitamin A from her everyday diet. Also, avoid using drugs and cosmetics that contain retinol, a form of Vitamin A used to cure acne and other skin problems.

7. **Excess Caffeine**

Intake of caffeine should be limited during pregnancy as it increases the risk of miscarriage and stillbirth. Moreover, caffeine can lead to heartburn, an irritating sensation between the throat and the stomach.

8. **Herbal Tea**

Avoid drinking herbal tea, even the ones recommended for pregnant women, as there are some herbs that act as unwanted drugs, causing side effects and defects in a growing fetus.

9. **Alcohol**

Avoid alcohol completely during pregnancy, as drinking alcohol, no matter the amount, causes higher risks of miscarriage and stillbirth. Alcohol affects the normal development of the baby, resulting in fetal alcohol syndrome, heart problems, mental retardation and low birth weight. Even moderate drinking will affect the baby's brain development.

10. **Unpasteurized Juice**

Eat fresh fruits instead of juices as fruits contain fiber essential to keep constipation away. Homemade juices are safe, but avoid consuming unpasteurized juices as they contain harmful bacteria.

Bonus Book

Understanding Postnatal Depression

Table of Contents:

Introduction

It may be one of the most difficult things to deal with and the most unexpected. Post-natal depression is one of those medical conditions that few understand. Not only does this tend to catch many women off guard, but even doctors aren't always pre-pared to help. There is so much wonderful anticipation of a baby arriving, and when that moment comes, many women expect to feel nothing but joy. As with any other aspect of pregnancy or parenthood however, there are often some rather unexpected elements that come up and that must be faced.

It's important to note that this is a very serious health condition and should be ad-dressed appropriately. Though postnatal depression used to be quite misunderstood and therefore misdiagnosed, it is taken very seriously within the medical community. You need to discuss this condition with a doctor, even during your pregnancy, so that you understand the symptoms.

This isn't something that happens to "other women;" this is a condition over which you have no control and for which there is a great deal of help available. So, though you may feel as if this condition is something to feel bad about, this is a very common condition for which you can receive a great deal of help.

The problem is that it hits many women without warning. Just as a woman feels that she is finally able to embrace this new chapter in her life and love and adore her new little bundle, the hormones and emotions take over. This is very frustrating and dis-heartening and may even be brushed off, because most women want to believe that this can't possibly happen to them.

The reality is that many women feel depression on varying levels.Therefore, the time to move forward and determine if there is something going on is right away. You can get help; you can get back to normal, and you can enjoy your new little baby. How-ever, you have to first recognize what exactly is going on. That's often the hardest part—admitting that something is wrong in the first place!

We are going to take you through a journey and discuss what to be on the lookout for. We are going to help you to understand the steps, the symptoms, and how to cope with it all. This isn't something to be taken lightly, and, though it affects women on varying levels, postnatal depression is something for which you should prepare, just in case it happens to you.

Let's start by recognizing that this condition doesn't mean that there's anything wrong with you as a mother. This has nothing to do with your amount of love or adoration for your newborn. This condition has everything to do with your hormones, your body adjusting to birth, and life after birth with a newborn. It can even come on due to lack of sleep or nutrients or other basic fundamental needs. Knowing this in advance can really help you to feel prepared and to cope with the situation, if you are, in fact, somebody that suffers from postnatal depression.

Know, too, that not everybody feels the effects of this in the same way. You may know of a friend or family member who had a very mild case where she felt a bit sad or blue and that was the end of it. You may even know of somebody on the other end of the spectrum, who struggled and spent months feeling bouts of crying and even anger. Just know that no two cases are the same and you should be prepared for the unexpected.

You may go through your pregnancy with ease and then find that the months after baby's arrival are the most difficult. You may make it through the first few months with nothing at all. If nothing else, there must be greater awareness for postpartum depression and so this book will help to highlight what to know and how to get the help that you may find that you need.

Understanding Postnatal Depression

One of the biggest problems with postnatal depression is understanding it. This is a condition that, for many years, was misdiagnosed or ignored because the medical community and society, in general really didn't have the knowledge required to help. Many women suffered through the symptoms and depression, and it made for a very rough transition into motherhood. The sadness was confused with an adjustment period, and doctors and even friends and family just stood by while women suffered.

Fortunately, there is so much more information out there about postnatal depression now. This has become such a commonly observed condition that many doctors discuss the symptoms and likelihood of postnatal depression with their patients during pregnancy.

It's often hard for people to understand why postnatal depression occurs. The birth of a child is supposed to be such a positive and wonderful experience. Some women wait their whole lives for this or go through difficulties in conceiving, and, so, it doesn't seem natural that they are filled with sadness after the birth occurs. Many don't want to believe it and, therefore, the misconceptions and bad information tend to come to the forefront.

No woman wants to go through postnatal depression, but it is more common than you might realize. Just as no pregnancy is the same, no postnatal period is the same either. Even with your own pregnancies, you may suffer from absolutely no symptoms at all with one pregnancy and then find yourself lost in the depths of depression with your next. So, know that you are not alone, and that many women have gone through the same sentiments and symptoms from which you suffer. To some that offers comfort alone and therefore an understanding of what this health condition is all about.

Getting to the Heart of the Issue

We'll discuss the ins and outs of postnatal depression, but, first, there must be an understanding of the condition itself. Knowing what it's all about can help you to be aware of it and recognize if you are going through it. Some women find that being prepared for the potential onset for postnatal depression can be of great help in this already transitional time period of their lives. Some important things to know about postnatal depression include:

It often starts with a feeling of sadness: Though you are feeling hormonal and exhausted you may blow off your feelings of sadness. This is very common because most women don't want to believe that they feel sad during a seemingly happy time. Though a bit of sadness may be nothing, this is often the first sign and something to watch. If the sadness continues or worsens, then it may be necessary to get some help or to talk to your doctor.

It can be confused with a lack of sleep or difficulty adjusting: Sure you are going through a major transition in your life and that's all normal. The problem arises, however, when you are exhausted, have a difficult time in adjusting, can't seem to bond with the baby, or are feeling sad more often than not. If you are feeling hopeless or find that the adjustment is more than you can handle or that you even anticipated, then that's when it is likely that you are suffering from some level of postnatal depression.

It is usually present within the first few months after the baby arrives, but can be present for a year afterwards: What many people don't realize is that the symptoms of postpartum depression can come on and linger for over a year after baby arrives. This means that you may be suffering months after the arrival and have the symptoms and not even realize it.

Many women don't want to admit what they are feeling or don't ask for the help that they need: There is no shame whatsoever in admitting that you feel the symptoms of this. As a matter of fact it's admirable to get help and it is very common. So, you must recognize that if sadness or even hopelessness is present or if you are having a hard time bonding with baby or can't stop crying, you need help. Postpartum depression is a very real medical condition and must be diagnosed properly to allow the woman to get back to normal.

Why Does This Occur?

So as you work to understand what postnatal depression is all about, you may wonder to yourself why this occurs in the first place. It seems almost unnatural or at least unfair: How can a woman wait so long to enjoy her baby and then be overcome with sadness? This is a question that many women have asked and few have found the real answers to. The truth is that though there are very reasonable explanations, it just doesn't make sense in terms of fairness.

This is one of those medical conditions for which there may be no reasonable explanation. Sure, certain factors -- such as genetics, history, and even lifestyle -- can play into it, but this is not true all the time. Though you may feel hopeless or helpless for an explanation, it may be beneficial to just accept this condition for what it is and then to move on to getting the help that you need. .

You might feel as if the factors behind t apply to you, but they may be present even without your realizing it. So, in terms of awareness, you do want to investigate which ones make sense or apply and which ones do not. Think through your current situation, even during pregnancy, and then gain the necessary understanding to see why postpartum depression comes on.

Every woman is different; every pregnancy is different, and every instance of postnatal depression is different. A big part of understanding it, however, is to gain insight as to why it may occur. Remember that this isn't necessarily the same for everyone, but the reasons highlighted here are quite common. Though your situation may be different than somebody else who suffers from postnatal depression, some of these reasons may be present even if you don't realize it at the time.

Insight as to What Causes This to Occur

Awareness is everything with this condition and so looking at some of the most common reasons may help. Though these are just a few they do happen to be the most common. Do talk to your doctor if you have any concerns and if you are worried because these apply to you before pregnancy. Then be sure to know what you should be on the lookout for.

Change in hormone levels: This may be the most identifiable reason. Hormone levels change drastically during pregnancy. After you have given birth and you are trying to get back to normal, the hormone levels are changing all over again. The changes may be extreme and may cause a woman to feel the effects, often exhibited through high highs and very low lows. So, know that the hormones that are changing and going crazy within you are very normal and may cause postpartum depression in the first place.

Caring for a sick or colicky baby: Those women who are caring for fussy or even colicky babies may find that they suffer from postnatal depression. As her entire focus is on a crying or needy infant, it is only natural that the mother may have a hard time coping. When you couple very trying and challenging days with fluctuating hormone levels, it often results in postnatal depression.

Already suffering from depression: A woman who already had depression, either during or even before pregnancy, may find that she is more prone to postpartum depression. She already suffers from the feelings of sadness and this is often complicated after the birth of a child. This is particularly true if the woman was on medication and has had to change that due to pregnancy.

Stress or other medical conditions present in life: If a woman is suffering from other forms of stress or other medical conditions, it may mean that she is more likely to develop postnatal depression. It is often hard to cope with these matters and, when you add to it the fact that she may also be sleep deprived or not able to care for her, and then it can be a recipe for disaster. It is often difficult to cope with this and, just a bit of stress can send a woman over the edge.

Why Is This Condition So Often Ignored or Misdiagnosed?

Though this condition has become more common than it ever used to be, there is still a lack of awareness or education. Even the most educated doctor may struggle to recognize or even diagnose the symptoms of postnatal depression, particularly if they are a bit subtler in nature. Awareness is a bit part of this, not only for pregnant women, but also for the medical community as a whole.

There are, of course, the telltale signs but sometimes they may not present in the same way. The women who feel more subtle signs are often at a loss and therefore may find difficulties in getting the help that they need. Not only is there often a difficulty in diagnosing the problem, but there may also be a difficulty in detecting what is happening. It must start with the woman specifically, as she must be in tune with what is going on within her and be forthcoming about it.

So, it may begin with a lack of awareness or an inability to really admit what is going on. Again, this is nothing to be ashamed of, though many women feel differently when they are going through it. This is very common and the only way to get help and to feel your normal self again is to determine what is going on and to pinpoint the symptoms that you are suffering from.

You want to be sure that you have a good doctor with whom you can have an open discussion, as that will be of the greatest help to you. So, start with the understanding and then recognize just why it is that this condition is so often ignored or improperly diagnosed. Here are just a few of the reasons why many women don't get the help that they need or realize that there is a problem at all.

A lack of awareness overall: Though there is far more information out there than there ever used to be, the truth is that there is still a general lack of awareness. Since this is not a typical medical condition or is something that many doctors aren't sure how to diagnose or treat, there is a great misunderstanding. That means that, as the lack of awareness goes on or education is missing, there are women who are suffering needlessly. Any attempts at building awareness are important, as they can help the medical community, as well as all of the women who are suffering from postnatal depression individually.

A feeling of shame or not wanting to believe this is true: Sometimes the problem comes from the woman specifically. She doesn't want to believe that this is happening and wants to pretend that she is okay, when really she is not. So in her shame or feelings of wanting to be positive, she tends to ignore the telltale signs or tell herself that she is okay. Even after going to a doctor's appointment she may be hesitant to tell her doctor what is happening, and so the problem goes undiagnosed as the woman isn't forthcoming of what she is feeling and going through.

A doctor not recognizing more subtle symptoms: A simple feeling of sadness may be nothing or it may be the start of postnatal depression specifically. A woman may feel anxious or overwhelmed and this may not be recognized as part of the condition when it really is. Though many women tend to think of sadness as the only symptom, there are others possible and present that may be part of the problem. These subtle symptoms aren't often recognized by the woman and may not even be recognized by the doctor either, and that's where the problem really starts.

A lack of education as to how to help a woman suffering from this condition: Though the condition may be recognized and even diagnosed, some doctors aren't sure how to help their patients. They may offer a pamphlet but no real support. It's imperative that women get the help that they need whether it's a support group, proper literature, coping mechanisms, or even psychiatric help if necessary. Though the problem may be recognized, it's not enough if she doesn't get the help that she really needs to cope with it and try to get back to normal. Help is needed and that's part of the awareness and education!

How Can a Happy Mother Suffer from This?

The thing to remember about postnatal depression is that this is not the norm, meaning the woman doesn't feel like herself. It may be easy to see from an outside perspective or it may be a bit more difficult, if the woman is trying to cover it up. Nevertheless, there is something that just feels off within the woman. It may be as obvious as nonstop crying bouts or it may be more subtle such as passing fits of anxiety, as the woman tries hard to adjust to her new lifestyle.

Having a baby is a huge transition and many women need time to cope with the new responsibilities and changes. Along with that can come a change in the woman's demeanor or mindset. It may feel as though a seemingly happy woman has absolutely no control over feeling sadness, frustration, anxiety, or just generally overwhelmed. When a usually happy woman starts struggling with these emotions you can see postpartum depression setting in and it turns an excited and hopeful individual into a withdrawn and overwhelmed one very quickly.

There is a great deal of blame on the mother's part and even others around her when it comes to the range of emotions. This is not a condition that any new mother would choose and so it should never be seen as a reflection of who the mother is or how great a caretaker she is. This is a true medical condition like anything else and therefore it should be taken seriously. No woman sets out to feel miserable or overly anxious after the arrival of her newborn child.

So, there needs to be sensitivity to this and a realization that these emotions are well beyond your control. This needs to start with the mother going through it and should filter out to all of those around her who love her and need to support her. Offering help or just being there for a woman suffering from postnatal depression may be the best thing that a loved one can do. Never judge or think that this is controllable—women want to enjoy their new babies and when they can't, there should be the realization that something isn't quite right!

Realizing That Something Is Amiss

Anybody who has gone through postnatal depression or knows of somebody who has can attest to the fact that this is a very difficult condition. So bear in mind that this is not a choice or a condition that somebody would ever want. Here are a few things to realize and help to show that this is not just a woman choosing to be unhappy or overwhelmed.

It has nothing to do with the mother's demeanor or happiness: Even if the mother wasn't a particularly positive person before, this condition has nothing to do with her demeanor afterwards. It is easy to see when an otherwise happy woman is suddenly sad and withdrawn after the birth of her child. The unfortunate thing to note, however, is that it is often more subtle than this. You may notice a change in demeanor, but even if you just think that something is off, it's worth asking about. Women suffering through postpartum depression often just want somebody to be there for them or to notice that something isn't quite right.

It doesn't mean that the mother doesn't love or appreciate her baby: There should be no confusing the symptoms of this condition with the notion that the mother doesn't love or care for her baby. The mother does love and care for her baby and wants to share that closeness more than anything. It is therefore important to realize this and to offer support, if you see a mother struggling with the rise and fall of these emotions and symptoms of postnatal depression.

The symptoms tend to take over the woman and control her feelings: Oftentimes a woman suffering from postnatal depression is experiencing things that are well beyond her own control. Therefore she can't stop the overwhelming roller coaster of emotions that she is experiencing even if she wants to. This can make a woman feel helpless particularly if all she has ever wanted to do was have a baby. She will get through this but does need support!

The mother should never feel bad about suffering from this medical condition, but should recognize a difference and get some help: This is truly a medical condition like anything else and should be treated as such. A woman suffering from this needs help, needs recognition of what is going on, and needs support and treatment. Though this will often subside with time, a woman in this situation needs medical attention and should be treated as a patient as that's the situation at hand. This is not something she can control and she would never choose this path for herself, so support is the very best thing to offer!

How to Diagnosis the Problem

Many women who have suffered from postnatal depression will tell you that diagnosis and detection is the hardest part. First and foremost many mothers are ashamed to admit that this problem exists. They are worried what others will think and truthfully don't want to admit it to themselves as it's very upsetting. Though this is a very common condition after a baby, many women have a hard time admitting that they are suffering from it. Though the telltale signs may be there, they don't want to admit that they are struggling and so diagnosis can be a major issue.

Even for the medical professionals or friends and family that support the woman in this situation, it can be rather difficult to work towards diagnosis. All too often the woman isn't being forthcoming about what is going on within her. Either that or the signs are too subtle to pick up on. Even a trained medical professional may miss the signs or may not necessarily be equipped to handle this condition. Therefore you see that diagnosis is often a very difficult part of the process and that's unfortunate since it's how things move forward and progress.

To get proper diagnosis, first and foremost the woman needs to be forthcoming about her condition. If she is feeling even a bit of sadness or anxiety then it's best to mention this to those who support her or to a doctor. It's imperative to get an evaluation and to get the help you need in order to make it past the hardest point of the process—the beginning. Therefore you see that the way in which a woman portrays her symptoms and talks about them is what will help her to get clarity and otherwise move forward with her life. It is crucial to be on the lookout for anything out of the ordinary and detect when perhaps something just isn't quite right.

A big part of diagnosis falls on the woman and her ability to be open and honest about what is going on. Additionally it's important to be educated when a new baby arrives on what can be happening within the mother in the process. Education is a big part of this and can really help to prepare women and their support networks for the types of changes that may occur and point to postpartum depression. This is an important part of the process and why learning what to look for can really help to propel a woman towards diagnosis and related treatment. The sooner this happens, the sooner the woman can get back to enjoying her baby and feeling her normal self!

So How Can Diagnosis Occur?

Knowing just how important diagnosis can be isn't enough. There is a necessity to be in tune to it and ready to move forward with the process. If you are the woman suffering through the symptoms then you must learn to be in tune with how you are feeling and what is going on within you. If you are somebody supporting a woman that is clearly going through it, then you need to be ready to jump in and help her however possible. Here are a few indicators and ways to move towards proper diagnosis and related next steps:

Look for differences in the overall demeanor: This may be the best indicator and most important way to move towards proper diagnosis. Though it may be subtle you can often look for some changes to the woman's demeanor. Sure she's tired and sure she's dealing with a lot of adjustment, but this takes things one step further and indicates that something is just a bit "off". This is easier to detect if the woman's personality is majorly altered but it's best to be on the lookout anytime something just seems out of the norm. A good conversation to find out what is going on may unveil that there are some major issues beneath the surface, which ultimately allows a woman to get some help.

Be aware of the changing hormone levels and reactions as a result of this: There is so much going on within a woman during pregnancy and we all recognize that. For some reason however there is a tendency to forget just how much is going on within a woman after the baby is actually born. This may be the time when most women need help more so than any other. The fluctuating hormones combined with the lack of sleep and adjustments that a woman is going through can set the stage for postpartum depression, often without her even realizing it. If that's the case then there must be an awareness and related compassion for the fact that this is a lot on a woman and therefore she needs help. This is something to be aware of and look for as the woman going through it or the loved ones surrounding her.

Look for difficulty in coping or even in bonding with the baby: If a woman seems to have a difficult time in coping with everyday life that may be an indicator. Another telltale sign is when a woman has a very difficult time in bonding with her baby. She may not seem interested in the baby, may seem frustrated with the baby, or may just seem to be withdrawn from the baby altogether. This is usually quite obvious but hard for people to admit because everybody wants to think that there is a natural bond that exists immediately between mother and child. Sometimes it just takes awhile for that bond to develop. Sometimes there is hesitancy for the mother to get close, particularly if there was some traumatic circumstance or if the baby is sick or colicky. Always ask for help or ask if there is something going on because that just might help the woman who can't figure out within herself exactly what is going on.

Be aware of the usual symptoms as well as the more subtle signs: A woman needs to stay in tune with what she is feeling. Those around her need to be aware of anything out of the norm. It may be as obvious as having a difficult time in bonding with the baby or it may be subtler like just feeling down. As different as the cases of postnatal depression are, so too are the signs of it. Sometimes a woman may just not feel like herself. Other times a woman may feel that she isn't a good mother. There are multiple variations on what postnatal depression can be and how it shows itself, but getting diagnosis and being in tune with what is going on is imperative.

Talk to a doctor: A woman must always talk to her doctor and be honest with what she is feeling. She must be forthcoming about her emotions, her difficulties in adjusting, and what she is thinking. Just getting this out and talking to somebody who can help is where diagnosis comes from. So though it may seem difficult, this is how you move forward. The only true way to get a proper diagnosis is to speak honestly, talk through what is going on, and get the help that you need from a trusted professional. This is how you break through the problem and get a woman in this situation the needed help so that she can move forward with her life.

The Various Stages or Variations of Postnatal Depression

Again it's important to note that no two cases of postnatal depression are the same. There are many elements that go into this condition and therefore the way that it shows through with each woman may vary significantly. Being in tune to the signs of postnatal depression can be an excellent way to detect when there may be an instance of this. Though you may follow a different path or may suffer through the condition differently or silently, you should know how it usually evolves.

The following are very typical signs of how postnatal depression may occur. Again sometimes it may just be to the first stage and then go away as fast as it came on. The more extreme cases may go through all of these signs and even more time and time again. Just understanding what the typical stages are is a great start and then you can determine how exactly it is evolving within you and what you can do to get help for it. So here are the typical stages of postnatal depression and how they tend to show themselves on the average.

1. **Denial:** This is often where things get started off poorly as most women truly don't want to admit that something is wrong. It's much easier to just deny that the symptoms are there and pretend that everything is normal. No new mother wants to feel at a loss for bonding with her baby or feeling that sense of closeness. No new mother wants to feel isolated or detached from reality. So it only makes sense that denial is a big part of this and therefore why it's the first and most common stage of the process.

2. **Anger:** You might not think of this as a common stage of postnatal depression but it often is. A woman feels a huge sense of anger that she is suffering through anything but pure happiness. She feels frustrated, bitter, and very upset that these first few weeks after baby are far less than she ever expected. She feels mad at herself, mad at the situation, and in some cases may even feel mad at the baby as well.

3. **Depression:** This is often where we see things come out the most often with postnatal depression. The woman feels a sadness, sometimes uncontrollable through crying fits and an overall sadness that appears often. The depression may come and go or may linger, causing it to interfere with her daily life. Depression is a part of the name and so you know and recognize that it's also a part of the process as well. The depression may be even more intense if the woman suffered from depression before pregnancy or if the baby is very difficult to care for such as through illness or fussiness.

4. **Acceptance:** This is where many hope that women end up with in the process of

postpartum depression. There is a hope that the woman learns to accept this condition, but that often comes only after proper diagnosis and the help that she needs. Therefore acceptance may not always be as readily available as most would hope for and it takes time to get there. This often won't come about until a woman can figure out what is going on and learn how to get back to her normal self.

What Are the Variations Involved?

The symptoms may vary, the stages may vary, and so too may the actual stages as well. Knowing that it's important to recognize that the variations may be subtle or extreme, with a real hope that there is help for those that ever get towards the more extreme phases. Therefore you should know that these stages may go through sequence or may come on at a more severe degree with no warning. Either way, these should all be treated carefully and should be indicators that something is just not right.

Here are the most common variations of postpartum depression:

Sadness: This may be just a feeling of being "down in the dumps" or show forth as a real depression in its truest form. This may come through as a first sign or may linger as the most pressing symptom that a woman ever gets. Whatever the case things tend to start with sadness and that may be an underlying aspect of things moving forward.

Anxiety and Feeling Overwhelmed: In addition to the very natural parts of feeling exhausted and even stressed due to the new adjustment in her life, a woman may feel full of anxiety. This may come about due to feeling overwhelmed or exist independently. Though the woman may try to adjust and to cope with these unexpected feelings, she often can't learn to deal with them clearly and they often get the best of her.

Being Withdrawn: The woman may seem to be withdrawn from her friends and family, withdrawn from everyday life, or even withdrawn from her baby. She may seem to be sort of in a shell and have a difficult time in finding happiness or learning to adapt to this new chapter of her life. She may have difficulty in coping and in functioning and therefore feel that withdrawing from everyone and everything close to her makes for a much more palatable situation.

Full Depression and Difficulty in Coping or Functioning: The first few variations are a bit subtler but this one is very obvious. The woman seems unfocused, is very clearly depressed, and often has a hard time in just dealing with anything.

She is sad, may cry a lot, and may also seem angry, overwhelmed, and anxious. She can't cope with the new role of motherhood and may also have a difficult time in figuring out how to make things work in her life. She may feel isolated, alone, and as if she is going through this all on her own. She may have crying fits or just walk around in a fog most of the time, having a hard time even concentrating or holding a conversation.

Psychosis or More Serious Mental Health Issues: This is the most extreme of the variations. The woman that has a difficult time in even getting out of bed. She is completely out of sorts and this often occurs if she suffered with depression or mental health issues before pregnancy, but that's not always the case. She is completely outside of herself, often wants nothing to do with the baby, and is clearly disturbed to the point of concern from her loved ones. This is not the "norm" but should be taken very seriously by those that care for her as some help is needed.

Everyone is different but these stages and variations can help to provide a guideline to show what postpartum depression is and how it shows itself. Even the more minor or subtle cases require some intervention and help, because no woman wants to suffer with this. Therefore all cases should be taken seriously and a woman should always be offered proper diagnosis and help whenever possible.

Getting Help for the Mother Who Needs It

We've seen by now that diagnosis is one of the most important aspects of postnatal depression. Recognizing the problem is the only surefire way to get the mother the help that she truly needs. The identification of the problem and therefore the related process required to help the mother are an important first step in the process. Though you may think that a mother easily recognizes her own symptoms and can get herself the help that she needs, this may not always be the case.

What you must recognize about this condition is that not only does the mother have a hard time recognizing it or coming clean about it, but she also isn't sure of where to turn for help. Even if she identifies that she is struggling with postnatal depression and wants to help herself, she often doesn't know where to turn or what to do next. This is a terrible and often isolating feeling for a mother who so desperately wants to enjoy her new role. It's bad enough that the mother is having a hard time adjusting and trying to reclaim normalcy but she may often struggle in silence for fear of asking for help or simply not knowing where to turn. This happens all too often!

As education and awareness are an important part of the process, so too is the necessity to help mother through this difficult time. She may simply need to know that all is well and that she has somebody or some avenue that can get her heading in the right direction. This may come from a doctor, another trusted professional, or simply from her own support group of friends and family. No matter what the support that she receives, this plus any required treatment plan is what will help her to regain her strength and to feel once again as though she is able to adjust and enjoy her new baby.

So helping the mother becomes critical and it can happen in a variety of different ways. It's imperative that mother knows that she has people to turn to, that this is all normal and common, and that she will get help so that she can get back to normal and enjoy her new life. This is as important as the education behind postnatal depression and can ensure that a new mother never has to suffer in silence or feel alone again. Getting help to the mother becomes a critical way of moving forward and making postnatal depression a very livable condition for all involved.

Figuring Out How to Help a Woman through This Condition

As different as the actual condition postnatal depression may appear in women so too are the personalities and situations of the women who suffer from it. Therefore this is no such thing as a quick fix or as a "one size fits all" type of solution. Knowing that and recognizing that means that you must focus on these various tips and ensure that you help a woman in the most effective way possible for her.

Mother needs to know that this is very common and face her condition head on: Though mother may not want to face the facts she is going to have to in order to move forward with getting treatment. Knowing that there may be a necessity to get some help to mother in various forms. You may have to help point out to her that what she is feeling isn't necessarily normal and that postnatal depression is very common and very treatable. Ultimately the realization must come from the mother herself but she must also get a bit of encouragement and advice and insight from those that can lead her down the path to treatment.

There must be a proper support network in place: A mother is going to need her support network for a variety of reasons. She may need her closest and most trusted friends and family to help her to see what is going on or simply to talk to. She may need this support network to get advice from or to help her through a particularly bad day. If the baby is sick or fussy then she may even need help in caring for the baby at times. She may just need a break and turning to somebody for help in caring for the baby or for herself is going to be instrumental in her treatment. One should never underestimate the magnitude of a support network, particularly to a woman who is suffering from this condition in her everyday life.

Get help from a doctor, professional, or support group: In many instances it's not just enough to have the help from a friend or family member. In addition a woman may want to talk to her doctor about her symptoms and how she is coping. She may need treatment in the form of medication in some cases. She may need to speak to a trained professional like a psychiatrist if the problem is severe in nature. She may even need to join a local support group that is equipped in helping women who suffer from postnatal depression. No matter what, she needs to discuss her symptoms with a doctor to determine if there is any way to offer her the help that she needs. In most instances, a woman may not need medication or may even outgrow the need for it as she moves forward, but it's always wise to get the insight and help from a trained professional just in case.

Conclusion

Postnatal depression is a problem to be taken very seriously. No matter how minimal the symptoms may seem, this is a condition that can be devastating to live with. This is a condition for which much hasn't been known in the past but that is changing due to some long overdue education and awareness building. So as awareness is a big component in getting a woman help, this is a very positive change in the long run. Though there is still so much more that must be learned about postnatal depression, this is a condition for which more and more women are getting the help that they need due to proper education.

It is wise for women to become informed about postnatal depression even while they are pregnant. It doesn't necessarily mean that they will suffer from it or that they should be worried, but it's always wise to be prepared for anything. Therefore more and more doctors are taking steps to tell women what to look for in a proactive measure. This is great news for a condition for which many women have suffered through unnecessarily. Therefore the proper education behind this goes to show just how common this medical condition has come to be in recent years.

Though women may assume that the first few months or even year of baby's life are going to be filled with pure joy, sometimes they suffer from symptoms that they never anticipated. When you think about the change in hormones, the huge adjustment, the sleep deprivation, and the combination of all of these factors, it is no wonder that many women suffer from this condition and why it has become so common. The hormones alone can make for a very difficult situation as most women simply aren't sure of how to cope or how to express their feelings of anxiety and even depression.

It's important that women know that postnatal depression is common and that there is help for it. Since it was misunderstood and therefore misdiagnosed in the past it is no wonder that many women suffered in silence and isolation. These days there are so many ways to help a woman through this condition so that she can get back to enjoying her new role as mother.

It's important to be aware of the symptoms and to be on the lookout for the subtle and more obvious symptoms. Diagnosis and identification are difficult parts of the process, but imperative ones if a woman hopes to get back to her normal self.

Women with this condition need love and support and may need more depending on their particular situation. If the baby is sick or fussy then they may need even more support as they struggle to help their baby and care for themselves. This is a condition for which it may strike each woman differently. Therefore some symptoms may be subtler such as a minor sadness, while other symptoms may be more obvious such as crying fits.

No symptom should be taken lightly and it's therefore important to reach out to a new mother to do a sense check and make sure that all is right with her. Postnatal depression may be very common but it is a condition for which a woman needs help. Be aware as a mother of young children of what to look for and be there to support others that may be going through the symptoms. That is how you help to ensure that postnatal depression becomes a manageable condition and how we help more and more women through it each and every day.

Learning what this condition is all about, being aware of the possible symptoms, and recognizing that it may be different in every woman are the types of things and steps for which a woman will learn to live with this condition and enjoy her new role of mother—there is help and it starts here with learning all about the condition and how to make it more manageable in everyday life!

Thank You!

Printed in Great Britain
by Amazon.co.uk, Ltd.,
Marston Gate.